ROZA KAY

Atkins Diet Cookbook 2023

Budget -Friendly Low- Carb Meals

Contents

1 INTRODUCTION   1

    Knowing the Atkins Diet for People on a Tight Budget   1

    The Atkins Diet: A Basic Overview   1

    Myths Regarding the Atkins Diet's Cost   2

2 CHAPTER ONE   6

RECIPES FOR BREAKFAST   6

Recipe for Scrambled Eggs with Spinach and Feta   7

    Recipe for Greek Yogurt Parfait with Berries   10

    Recipe for Avocado and Bacon Breakfast Wraps   13

3 CHAPTER TWO   16

LUNCH IDEAS   16

    RECIPE FOR TUNA SALAD LETTUCE WRAPS.   17

    BROCCOLI AND CAULIFLOWER SOUP   20

    RECIPE FOR CHICKEN CAESAR SALAD   23

4 CHAPTER THREE   27

DINNER DELIGHTS   27

    RECIPE FOR ZUCCHINI NOODLES WITH PESTO   28

    RECIPE FOR BAKED SALMON WITH LEMON AND DILL   32

    RECIPE FOR MEATBALLS AND SQUASH   35

5 CHAPTER FOUR   40

SNACKS AND SIDES   40

    RECIPE FOR ROASTED BRUSSEL SPROUTS WITH PARMESAN   41

    RECIPE FOR CUCUMBER AND CREAM CHEESE ROLL-UPS   44

    AVOCADO WITH VEGETABLE STICKS   48

6 CHAPTER FIVE   52

    BUDGET-FRIENDLY DESSERTS   52

RECIPE FOR CHOCOLATE AVOCADO MOUSSE   53
RECIPE FOR BERRY CHIA SEED PUDDING   57
RECIPE FOR KETO-FRIENDLY PEANUT BUTTER COOK-
IES   61
7 CHAPTER SIX   65
MEAL PLANNING AND SHOPPING TIPS   65
Cost-effective Atkins Diet Shopping Techniques   67
8 CHAPTER SEVEN   70
Budget-Friendly Ingredient Swaps   70
How to Maximize Remaining Food   73
9 CONCLUSION   76
Your Path to Atkins Living on a Budget   78

1

INTRODUCTION

Knowing the Atkins Diet for People on a Tight Budget

Many people have adopted the popular low-carb Atkins Diet because it promises to aid in weight loss and enhance general health. There's a prevalent misperception that adhering to the Atkins Diet has to be costly, even though it can be beneficial in reaching these objectives. It is feasible to eat great, healthful meals and adhere to the Atkins Diet on a budget. The purpose of this chapter is to explain the Atkins Diet in plain English and show you how to make it affordable.

The Atkins Diet: A Basic Overview

Dr. Robert Atkins developed the Atkins Diet, which revolves around cutting less on carbohydrates to help the body switch from utilizing fat stores for energy to using glucose as its main source. It is frequently split into *four stages:*

The most restrictive phase, known as the **induction phase**, limits daily carbohydrate intake to about 20−25 grams. It seeks to induce ketosis, a state in which the body burns fat for energy.

Phase of Balancing: During this stage, you gradually increase your daily carbohydrate consumption to determine the precise amount of carbohydrates you need to lose or maintain weight.

Pre-Maintenance Phase: To get ready for maintenance, you raise your carb consumption as you get closer to your target weight.

Phase of maintenance: During this time, you keep your weight in check by eating a balanced diet and controlling your intake of carbohydrates.

Myths Regarding the Atkins Diet's Cost

A common misperception is that the Atkins Diet is pricey by nature. This misconception frequently results from the idea that foods high in protein and low in carbs are expensive. That need not be the case, though. This is the reason why:

Real Foods: Whole, real foods including meat, fish, eggs, and non-starchy vegetables are the focus of the Atkins Diet. These things are frequently available for fair pricing.

Reduced Requirement for Processed Foods: Conventional low-carb specialty items, such as pasta or bread, can be pricey. The main Atkins diet recommends consuming these processed foods in moderation.

Decreased Snacking: You can feel less hungry in between meals when following the Atkins Diet, which could result in less snacking and financial savings.

Advice for Budget-Friendly Atkins Nutrition

Plan Your Meals: Making a grocery list and meal plan according to your budget will assist you in staying on track.

Purchasing non-perishable low-carb goods in bulk can result in a more economical buy, such as nuts, seeds, and canned salmon.

Utilize Leftovers Creatively: To cut down on food waste and save money, repurpose leftovers into new meals.

Make specials and Discounts a Priority: Shop for low-carb essentials like meat, poultry, and veggies, and take advantage of specials and discounts.

Grow Your Own: To cut expenses, try cultivating your low-carb veggies and herbs, if at all possible.

Investigate Inexpensive Proteins: Less expensive protein sources, such as ground beef or chicken thighs, can offer comparable nutrition to more costly cuts.

Low-Cost dishes: Seek out Atkins-friendly dishes that are within your budget and make use of inexpensive products.

Advice for Budget-Friendly Low-Carb Eating

Consuming a diet low in carbohydrates doesn't have to be costly. You may maintain financial stability while reaping the rewards of a low-carb lifestyle with some careful preparation and thoughtful decision-making. *To help you eat low-carb on a budget, consider the following advice:*

Make a Weekly Meal Plan: List the foods you will eat for breakfast, lunch, dinner, and snacks. Making effective grocery lists and resisting the urge to order takeaway or eat out are two benefits of planning.

Accept Real Foods: Give priority to complete, unprocessed foods. Lean meats, eggs, dairy, and fresh veggies are frequently more affordable than processed or prepackaged low-carb substitutes.

Invest in Bulk: To save money over time, buy non-perishable low-carb basics like canned products, nuts, and seeds in large quantities. Check online or at warehouse stores for deals.

Cook in Bulk: Make bigger batches of meals and freeze them into single servings. In the long term, this saves you money and time by decreasing waste.

Examine Frozen Vegetables: This is an affordable and practical choice. They have a longer shelf life and frequently retain more nutrients than their fresh counterparts.

Creatively Utilize Leftovers: Incorporate leftovers into fresh dishes. For instance, you may make chicken salad today using the roasted chicken from last night.

Make specials and Discounts a Priority: Shop for low-carb essentials like meat, poultry, and veggies, and take advantage of specials and discounts. To save money, think about purchasing produce that is in season.

Cook from Scratch: Low-carb goods that come prepackaged can be expensive. You may keep prices and ingredients under control when you cook from scratch. Discover how to prepare your low-carb dressings, sauces, and snacks.

Grow Your Own: If you have the time and space, you should think about cultivating your low-carb herbs and veggies. Produce grown at home can be quite economical.

Examine Inexpensive Proteins: Although premium types of meat might be pricey, there are less expensive but equally nutrient-dense alternatives including ground beef, chicken thighs, and pork shoulder.

Restrict Specialty Products: Specialty low-carb items, such as keto bread or pasta, might cost more. Eat less of them and concentrate on meals that are naturally low in carbs.

Meal prep: Set aside some time every week to prepare snacks and meals ahead of time. Being able to easily access low-carb options lessens the need to order expensive takeout or fast food.

Cost-effective Recipes: Seek out recipes that are specially made for low-carb, cost-effective cooking. There are lots of tasty and inventive options available that won't break the bank.

Portion Control: Consider the sizes of your portions. Even so, eating too much low-carb food might still be expensive. Adhere to the suggested portion sizes.

Buy Local and Seasonal: At fair rates, local farmers' markets can provide fresh produce that is in season. It also promotes regional agriculture.

Become Informed: Acquire knowledge about the nutritive content of various foods. You can use this information to make wise and economical decisions.

Recall that choosing healthier foods is just as important as cutting costs while following a low-carb diet. You don't have to break the bank to enjoy a healthy, low-carb meal with a little preparation and ingenuity.

2

CHAPTER ONE

RECIPES FOR BREAKFAST

Recipe for Scrambled Eggs with Spinach and Feta

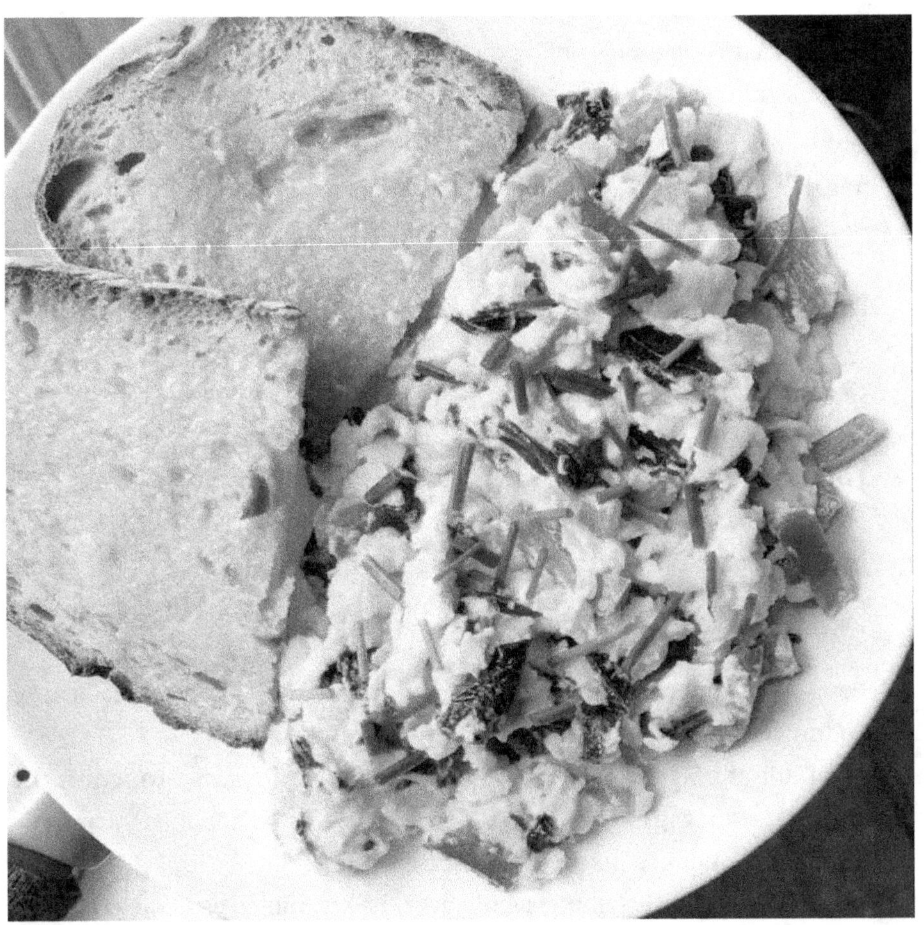

A tasty, low-carb meal that's quick and simple to make is scrambled eggs with spinach and feta. This recipe makes a filling breakfast by combining the tanginess of feta cheese, the earthy flavor of spinach, and the creaminess of eggs. This is how to prepare it:

For anyone following the Atkins Diet, this is an ideal quick and simple breakfast food. It has a lot of flavor, is low in carbohydrates and high in protein.

INGREDIENTS:

Two big eggs

One-third cup heavy cream
One tablespoon of butter.
1/4 cup of spinach, chopped
1/4 cup of feta cheese, crumbled
Add pepper and salt to taste.

INSTRUCTIONS:

- Get the ingredients ready: Once the yolks and whites of the eggs are thoroughly mixed, crack them into a basin and beat with a fork or whisk. Finely chop the fresh spinach and crumble in the feta cheese.
- Heat the Pan: Add the butter or olive oil to a nonstick skillet set over medium heat. Let it melt so that it coats the pan uniformly.
- Add the chopped spinach to the skillet and sauté it for one to two minutes, or until it wilts and gets soft.
- Pour the beaten eggs into the skillet containing the sautéed spinach after adding the eggs. Gently mix the eggs with the spinach.
- Scramble the Eggs: Keep cooking while using a spatula to whisk the mixture. Until the eggs are cooked to your preferred doneness, scramble them. This ought to take two to three minutes.
- Add Feta Cheese: Distribute evenly over the scrambled eggs the crumbled feta cheese. To mix the cheese into the eggs and let it to melt slightly, give it a quick stir.
- Add salt and pepper to taste when seasoning. Feta cheese can have a strong salt flavor, so use it with caution. It might not take much more salt.
- Serve: Spoon the scrambled eggs with spinach and feta onto a platter once the eggs are cooked through and the feta has melted somewhat.
- Optional Garnish: For a pop of color and flavor, you can choose to top your scrambled eggs with a sprinkling of fresh herbs like dill or parsley or a bit more crumbled feta.
- Have fun: You may now savor your scrambled eggs with spinach and feta. Savor the flavors—which are creamy, savory, and just a little tart—by serving them hot.

In addition to being tasty, this low-carb breakfast gives you a healthy amount of protein and nutrients to get your day started. Feel free to add extra flavor by customizing it with your preferred herbs or spices, as this recipe is rather adaptable.

TIPS:

Use full-fat cream cheese instead of heavy cream for a deeper taste.

For extra taste, add a pinch of paprika or nutmeg to the egg mixture.

For a full meal, serve with salsa or sliced avocado on the side.

NUTRITIONAL INFORMATION:

Serving size:half a cup

150 calories

12g of fat

2g of carbohydrates

12g of protein

Recipe for Greek Yogurt Parfait with Berries

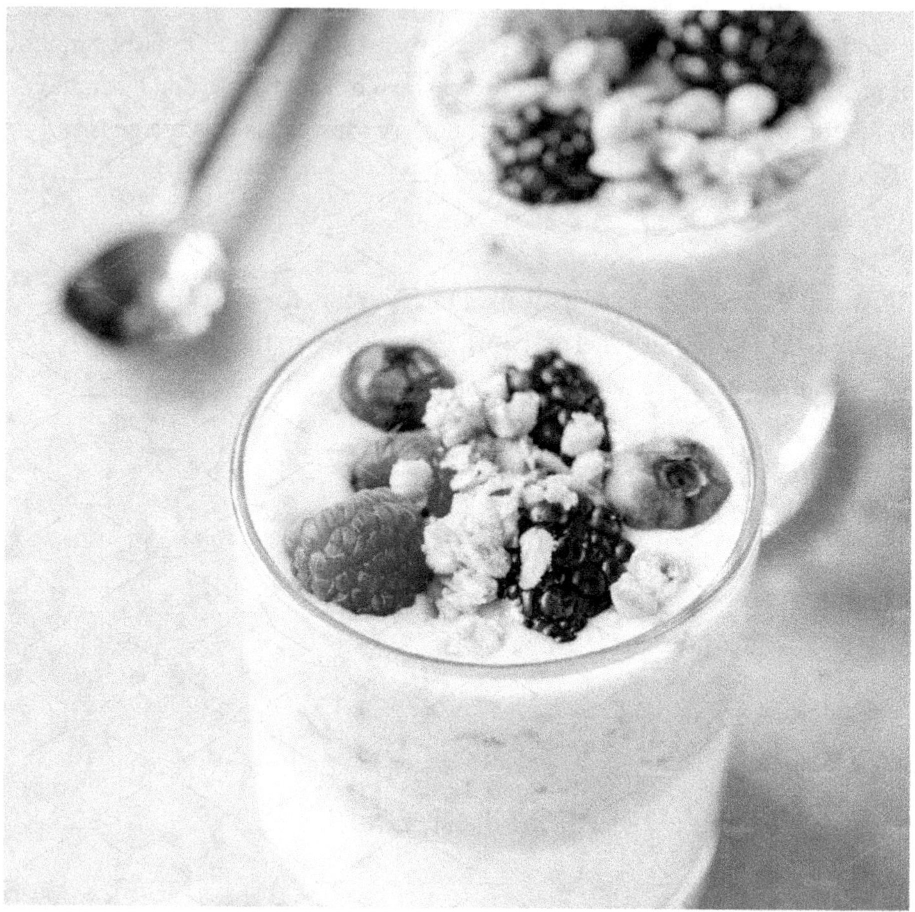

Berry-topped Greek yogurt parfaits are a tasty and healthy low-carb breakfast or snack choice. It's a wonderful delicacy that combines the sweetness of fresh berries with the richness of Greek yogurt. This is how to prepare it:

INGREDIENTS:

1 cup of plain Greek yogurt

Half a cup of fresh mixed berries, such as blueberries, raspberries, and strawberries

Two tablespoons of granola without sugar (optional)

One tablespoon of low-carb honey or sweetener (optional)

Garnish with fresh mint leaves (optional).

INSTRUCTIONS:

- Prepare Your Berries: Give your fresh mixed berries a thorough wash and rinse. For simpler layering, you can alternatively slice larger berries, like strawberries.
- Sweeten the Yogurt (Optional): You can pour honey or your preferred low-carb sweetener over the Greek yogurt if you'd like a little sweetness. Toss to blend well.
- Put the Parfait Together:In a clear glass or bowl, start with a layer of Greek yogurt at the bottom.
- Cover the yogurt with a layer of the fresh mixed berries.
- Sprinkle some of the granola, if using, on top of the berries. If you'd like, you may even top the yogurt and berries with another layer.
- Repeat Layers: Keep layering the ingredients until all of the berries and yogurt have been utilized. Don't forget to add a last layer of berries on top.
- Garnish (Optional): For a pop of color and extra freshness, you can choose to top your parfait with a sprig of fresh mint leaves.

It's time to serve your Greek yogurt parfait with berries. Savor it right now when the flavors are still vibrant and fresh.

TIPS:

Use more or less honey or sweetener to suit your taste in sweetness. For a lower-carb option, you can also leave it out completely.

Add more low-carb toppings to personalize your parfait, such as chopped nuts, seeds, or a touch of cinnamon.

Choose your granola carefully if you're following a strict low-carb or ketogenic diet, as many versions have additional sugars. If you're low on sugar, go for a granola made with nuts.

NUTRITIONAL INFORMATION:

Size of serving: 1 parfait

150 calories

Fat (5g)

10g of carbohydrates

20g of protein

In addition to being a delightful and fulfilling dessert, this Greek yogurt parfait with berries offers an excellent supply of protein, beneficial fats, and antioxidants from the berries. It's a fantastic way to savor a satisfying, low-carb breakfast or snack that leaves you feeling full and energized.

Recipe for Avocado and Bacon Breakfast Wraps

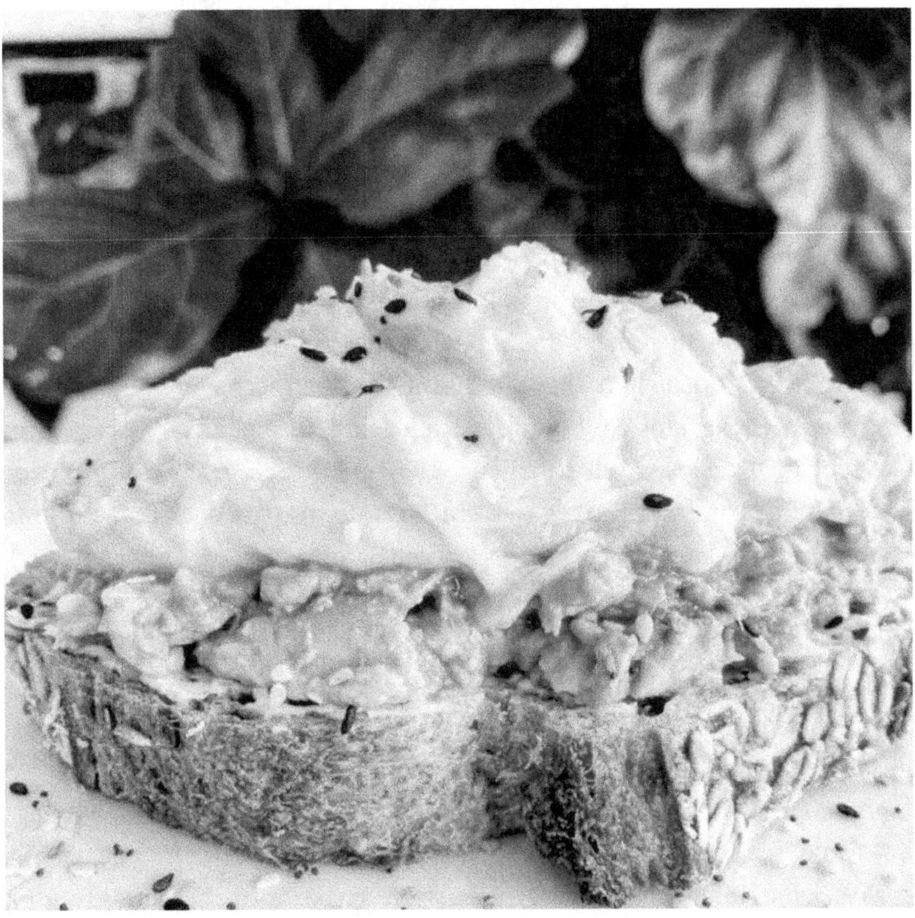

A tasty and filling low-carb breakfast option is an avocado and bacon breakfast wrap. It makes a tasty breakfast dish by fusing the smokey flavor of bacon with the creamy texture of avocado. This is how to prepare it:

INGREDIENTS:

One big avocado

Two to three cooked bacon pieces

Two big eggs

Add pepper and salt to taste.

For cooking, use oil or butter.

Low-carb tortilla or wraps made of lettuce

Toppings not required: fresh herbs, cheese, salsa, or hot sauce

INSTRUCTIONS

- Cook the Bacon: Allow the bacon to crisp up first. You can use the stovetop, oven, or microwave, whichever technique you like. When finished, cut the bacon into smaller pieces and set it on paper towels to drain any extra fat.
- Cut the avocado in half, take out the pit, and then scoop out the flesh into a basin. Using a fork, mash the avocado and add salt and pepper to taste.
- Cook the Eggs: Heat a little amount of oil or butter in a separate pan over medium heat. Once the eggs are cracked into the pan, cook them to your desired consistency (such as scrambled, sunny-side-up, or over-easy). Add salt and pepper to the eggs for seasoning.
- Build the Wrap:Arrange your lettuce leaves or low-carb tortilla on a sanitized surface.
- Transfer the mashed avocado onto the lettuce or tortilla.
- Top the avocado with the fried bacon slices.
- Transfer the cooked eggs to the layer of bacon.
- Top with extra Ingredients: You may personalize your wrap by adding extra ingredients like cheese, salsa, spicy sauce, or fresh herbs.
- Fold It Up: Gently fold the lettuce leaves or tortilla's sides over the filling. Then, to make your wrap, roll it up from the bottom.

It's time to serve your avocado and bacon breakfast wrap. Eat it as a quick breakfast or pack it in parchment paper for a dinner you can take with you.

Tips:

Depending on your diet constraints and personal inclination, you can make your wrap using either a large leaf of lettuce or a low-carb tortilla.

To improve the flavors, feel free to experiment with adding extras like diced tomatoes, onions, or a handful of shredded cheese.

Use full-fat cream instead of milk for a deeper taste.

For extra taste, add a pinch of cheese or herbs to the egg mixture.

For a full meal, serve with a side of fruit or vegetables.

This breakfast wrap is a fantastic low-carb or ketogenic option because of its amazing blend of flavors and textures. It's an easy and delicious way to have a filling breakfast every day.

NUTRITIONAL INFORMATION::
Size of serving: 1 wrap
250 calories
15g of fat
6g of carbohydrates
18g of protein

CHAPTER TWO

LUNCH IDEAS

RECIPE FOR TUNA SALAD LETTUCE WRAPS.

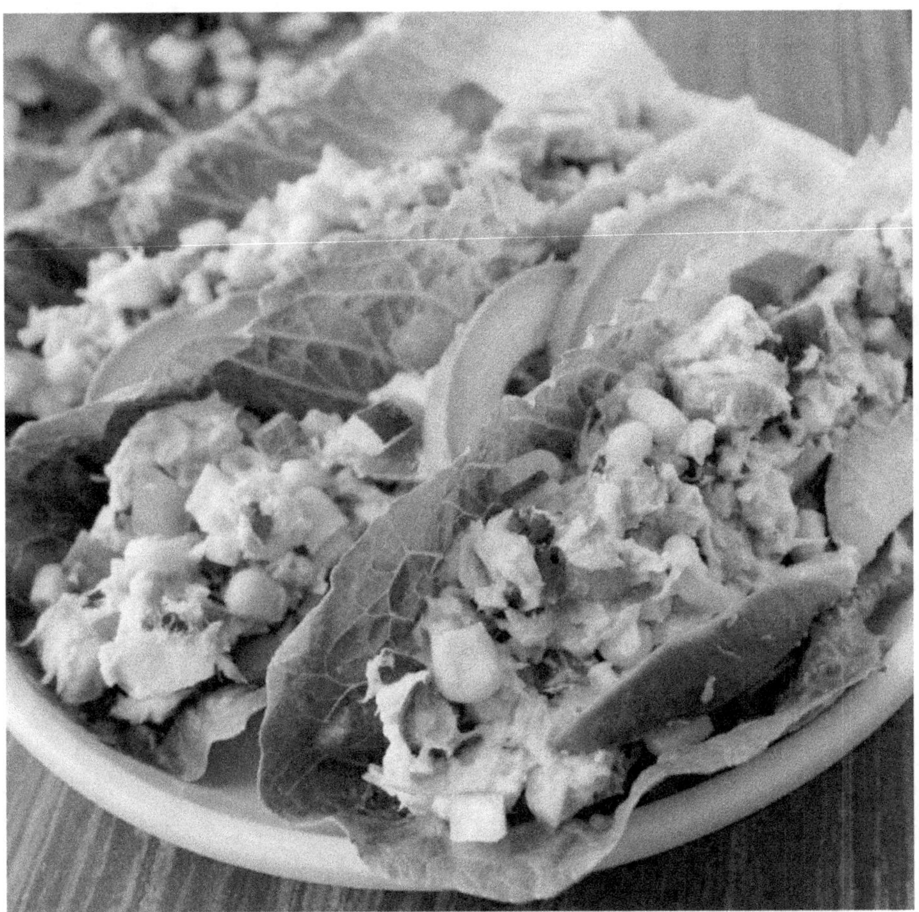

Fresh, healthful, and low-carb tuna salad lettuce wraps are a great substitute for classic tuna salad sandwiches. These wraps are ideal for a filling and light supper. This is how to prepare them:

INGREDIENTS:

One can (5 oz) of drained canned tuna in water

Mayonnaise, two to three teaspoons (adjust to your preferred creaminess)

1/4 cup celery, chopped finely

1/4 cup red onion, chopped finely

One-third cup lemon juice

Add pepper and salt to taste.

Lettuce leaves (such as Romaine or Iceberg) to wrap

Add-ons: sliced avocado, cucumbers, or tomatoes

INSTRUCTIONS:

Get the tuna salad ready by:

- The drained tuna, mayonnaise, red onion, celery, and chopped lemon juice should all be combined in a mixing dish.
- Mixing the components together ensures that everything is thoroughly mixed. To get the desired creaminess, adjust the mayonnaise.
- Season: To taste, add salt and pepper to the tuna salad. Because canned tuna might already be salty, use caution when adding salt.
- Put the Lettuce Wraps Together:
- Spoon a dollop of the tuna salad onto a lettuce leaf, centering it.
- You can choose to top the tuna salad with extras like avocado, cucumber slices, or tomato slices.
- Sum It Up: To make your lettuce wrap, gently fold the sides of the leaf over the filling and roll it up starting from the bottom.

It's time to serve your tuna salad lettuce wraps. Savor them as a light and revitalizing dinner.

Tips:

To enhance the flavor, sprinkle on some Dijon mustard or dill relish.

For a full meal, serve with a side of fruit or vegetables.

Replace the mayonnaise with full-fat for a richer tuna salad.

While any kind of lettuce will work for wrapping, the strong nature of iceberg and Romaine lettuces makes them ideal for holding the filling.

Try adding grated carrots, diced pickles, or bell peppers to your tuna salad for an added crunch.

You can add a touch of cayenne pepper or a dash of spicy sauce to the mixture if you want your tuna salad hotter.

Not only can tuna salad lettuce wraps be made quickly and deliciously as a light lunch or snack, but they are also low-carb and keto-friendly. They offer a filling mix of crisp, fresh vegetables and protein.

NUTRITIONAL INFORMATION:
Size of serving: 1 wrap
220 calories
15g of fat
3g of carbohydrates
25g of protein

BROCCOLI AND CAULIFLOWER SOUP

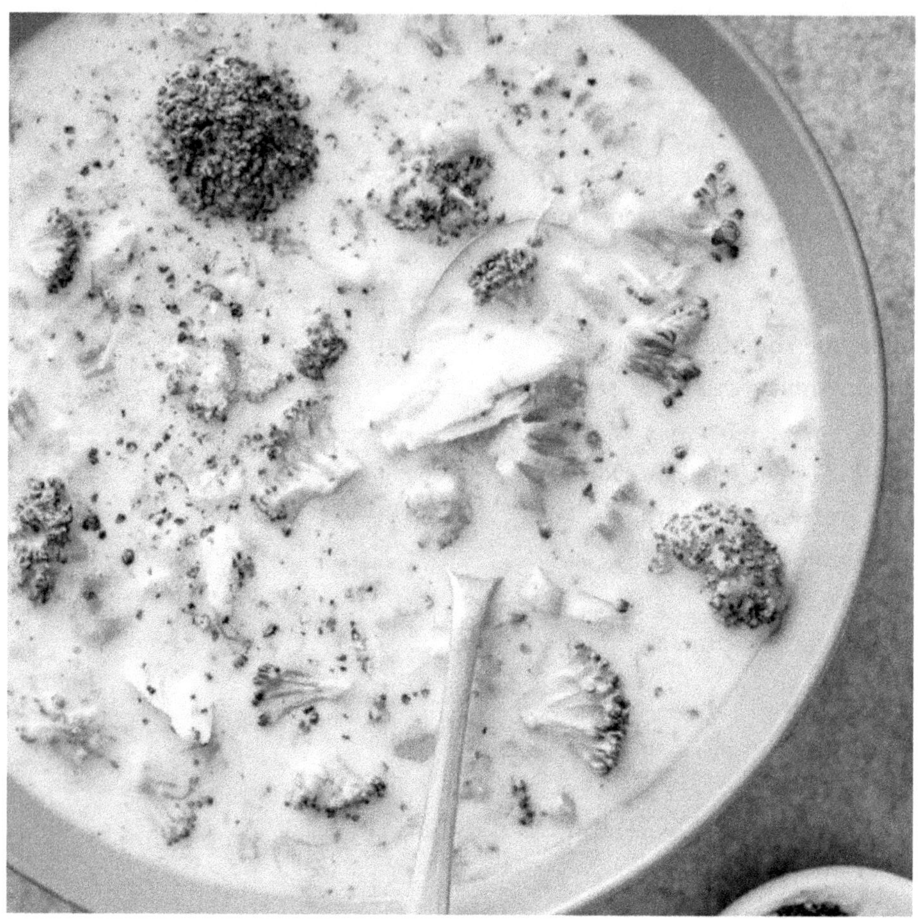

This is a tasty and nutritious soup that is ideal for people following the Atkins Diet. It is rich in nutrients, low in carbohydrates, and high in protein. It's a fantastic method to savor the tastes of these cruciferous veggies without going overboard on carbohydrates. This is how to prepare it:

INGREDIENTS:

One tiny cauliflower head, cut into florets

One tiny broccoli head, cut into florets

one sliced onion

two minced garlic cloves

Four cups of chicken or veggie stock

Half a cup of heavy cream, or, for a plant-based alternative, coconut cream

Two tablespoons of butter or olive oil

Add pepper and salt to taste.

Garnish with grated cheese, minced chives, or crispy bacon bits, if desired.

INSTRUCTIONS:

Get the veggies ready:

- Melt the butter or warm up the olive oil in a big pot over medium heat.
- Add the minced garlic and diced onion. They should be sautéed for a few minutes to turn transparent and tender.
- Add the broccoli and cauliflower florets to the saucepan. Let them caramelize slightly by sautéing them for approximately five minutes.
- Add the chicken or vegetable stock to the pot. Heat the mixture until it boils.
- Cover the pot and lower the heat to a simmer. Cook, stirring occasionally, until the veggies are soft, 15 to 20 minutes.
- Smooth and creamy soup can be achieved by blending it with an immersion blender or a conventional blender, working in batches if needed.
- Put the soup back on the low heat and blend in the coconut cream or heavy cream. To fully warm it through, let it boil for a few more minutes.
- Add salt and pepper to taste when preparing the soup. Always taste and adjust the seasoning to your liking.
- Pour the soups (carrot and broccoli) into individual bowls. If preferred, sprinkle on extras like crispy bacon bits, grated cheese, or minced chives.

Tips:

Lower the broth content or add more broccoli and cauliflower for a richer soup.

Use Parmesan cheese and full-fat heavy cream for a deeper taste.

You can add extra flavor to your soup by adjusting the seasoning with herbs or spices like paprika, thyme, or a dash of nutmeg.

You can save some of the cauliflower and broccoli florets before blending and then add them back into the soup if you would like it be chunkier.

Not only is this soup made of cauliflower and broccoli delicious, but it's also a great source of fiber and nutrients. It's a great low-carb alternative for a hearty and satisfying dinner.

NUTRITIONAL INFORMATION:
portion size: one cup
150 calories
12g of fat
5g of carbohydrates
10g of protein

Modifications:
Replace the heavy cream in this soup with coconut milk for a vegan version.

Add an additional 1/4 cup of heavy cream to make the soup creamier.

Add a splash of hot sauce or a pinch of red pepper flakes for more spiciness in your soup.

Add some cooked chicken or shrimp to the soup for a heartier dish.

Add some crumbled bacon or grated cheddar cheese to the soup for a unique flavor.

RECIPE FOR CHICKEN CAESAR SALAD

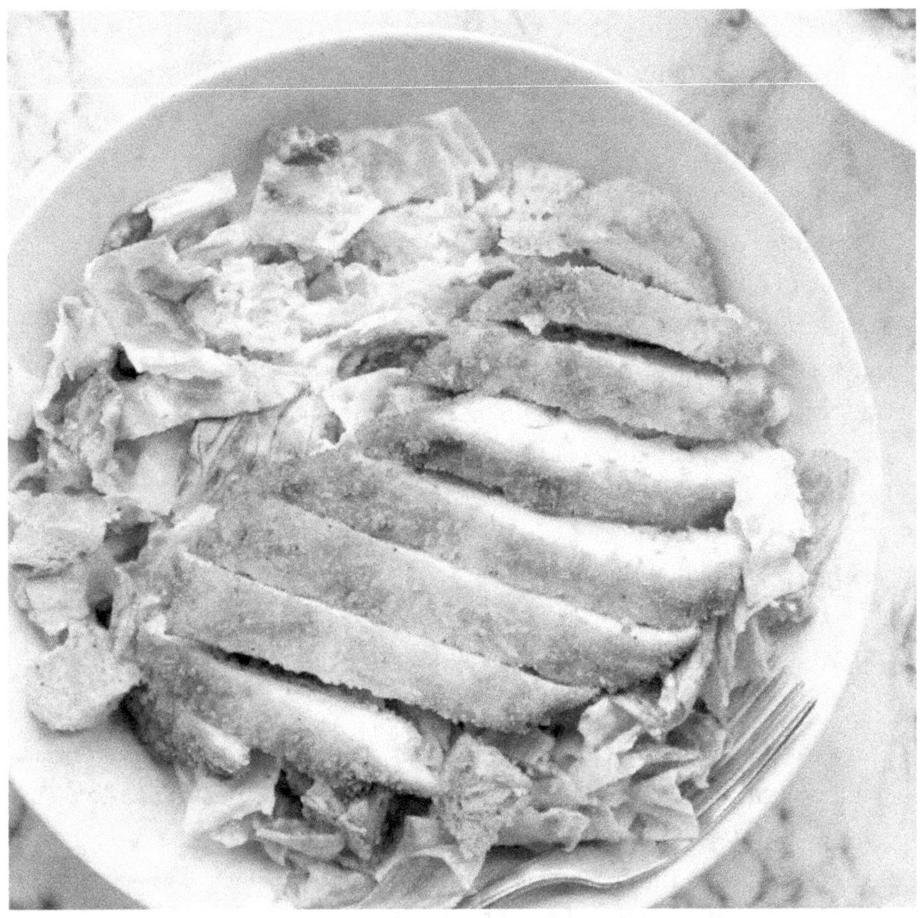

For a filling meal, a classic and delicious alternative is a chicken Caesar salad. This is how to prepare it:

INGREDIENTS:

For the Dressing of Caesar:

one-half cup mayonnaise

Grated Parmesan cheese, 1/4 cup; 2 tsp lemon juice

Two tsp Dijon mustard

two minced garlic cloves

One or two teaspoons of anchovy paste, or two anchovy fillets

To taste, add salt and black pepper.

Regarding Salad:

Two skinless and boneless chicken breasts

One tsp of olive oil

To taste, add salt and black pepper.

One sizable head of romaine lettuce, cleaned, and shredded into small pieces

One cup of handmade or store-bought croutons

For the topping, add more grated Parmesan cheese.

Lemon wedges, if desired, as a garnish

INSTRUCTIONS

Get the Caesar Dressing ready.

- Mix the mayonnaise, lemon juice, Dijon mustard, grated Parmesan cheese, minced garlic, and anchovy fillets (or three anchovy paste) in a bowl. To properly integrate the anchovies into the mixture, mash them in.
- Dressing Seasoning: Toss in a pinch of salt and black pepper to taste. Before using it, store it in the refrigerator.

Prepare the chicken:

- Turn the heat up to medium-high on a grill or grill pan.
- Add salt and pepper to the chicken breasts after brushing them with olive oil.
- When the chicken reaches an internal temperature of 165°F (75°C), grill it

for about 6 to 8 minutes on each side. The thickness of the chicken breasts will determine how long they take to cook.

· Cut the Chicken: After it's done cooking, give it a few minutes to rest. Next, cut it into bite-sized pieces or thin strips.

Put the Salad Together:

· Toss the croutons and shredded romaine lettuce together in a big bowl.
· Place the chicken slices over the salad.
· To season the salad, drizzle the chicken and salad with the Caesar dressing. Make sure the salad has an even coat of dressing by tossing it.

To serve, divide the salad (of chicken and Caesar) among different plates. If you'd like, add some more grated Parmesan cheese and lemon wedges as garnish.

Tips:
Store-bought croutons can be used, or toast bread pieces with a little olive oil and garlic to make your own.

You can also add extra toppings for extra taste and texture, such bacon bits, hard-boiled eggs, or cherry tomatoes.

To suit your taste, increase or decrease the amount of anchovies. Some people like their anchovies stronger, while others prefer them milder.

A timeless favorite, this chicken Caesar salad is made even better with homemade dressing. Savor it as a filling and healthy dinner.

NUTRITIONAL INFORMATION:
Size of serving: one salad
350 calories

15g of fat
15g of carbohydrates
35g of protein

4

CHAPTER THREE

DINNER DELIGHTS

RECIPE FOR ZUCCHINI NOODLES WITH PESTO

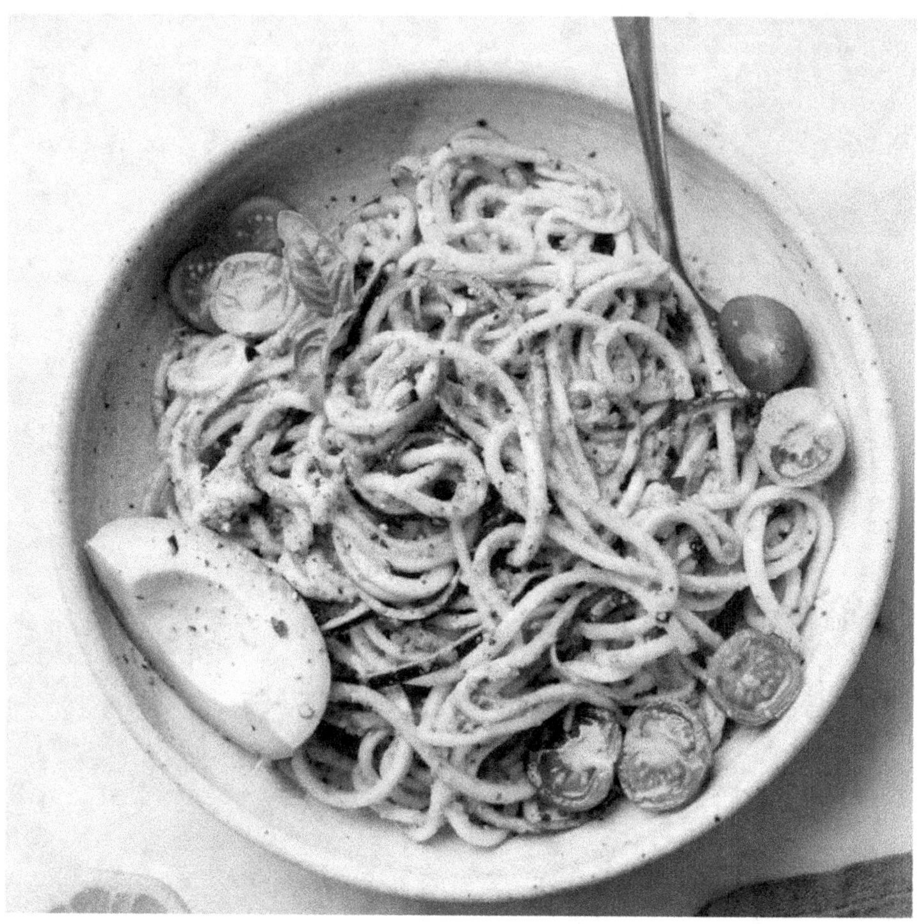

Pesto-topped zucchini noodles, sometimes known as zoodles, are a delicious and low-carb substitute for typical pasta meals. It has a lot of flavor, is low in carbohydrates, and high in protein. This is how to prepare it:

INGREDIENTS:

Regarding the Zucchini Soup:
   one or two medium zucchini
   Salted

Regarding Pesto:

two cups of newly packed basil leaves

Grated Parmesan cheese, half a cup

half a cup of walnuts or pine nuts

two minced garlic cloves

Half a cup of virgin olive oil

One-third cup of lemon juice

Add pepper and salt to taste.

Optional:

grated Parmigiano Reggiano

Halves of cherry tomatoes, roasted pine nuts

INSTRUCTIONS:

Get the zucchini noodles ready:

- Spiralize, julienne peel, or cut the zucchini into noodles with a knife. When using a spiralizer, adhere to the guidelines provided by the manufacturer.
- Zoodles can be placed on paper towels or in a colander. After giving them a light dusting of salt, leave them alone for ten to fifteen minutes. This aids in getting rid of extra moisture. After that, use paper towels to pat them dry.

Get the pesto ready:

- Grated Parmesan cheese, minced garlic, pine nuts (or walnuts), and fresh basil should all be combined in a food processor.
- Slowly sprinkle in the extra virgin olive oil while processing until the mixture is fully blended and silky.
- Add salt and pepper to taste when preparing the pesto. To get the desired amount of seasoning, adjust.

Put Together the Dish:

- Toss the freshly created pesto with the zucchini noodles in a big dish to coat them evenly.

To serve, divide the pesto-topped zucchini noodles among individual dishes. Add toasted pine nuts, sliced cherry tomatoes, and grated Parmesan cheese over top, if desired.

Advice:

If you like your zucchini noodles warm or slightly softened, you can sauté them for a minute or two in a pan with a little olive oil.

For more taste and protein, feel free to add grilled chicken, shrimp, or cherry tomatoes to your zoodle dish.

In a dry pan, toast the walnuts or pine nuts for a few minutes, or until they start to smell aromatic and gently brown. Their flavor is enhanced by this.

In addition to being low in fat and calories, zucchini noodles with pesto provide a taste explosion of bright, fresh aromas. Savor this recipe as a filling and light supper.

NUTRITIONAL INFORMATION:

portion size: one cup
150 calories
12g of fat
5g of carbohydrates
10g of protein

Modifications:

Use vegan pesto to make this dish vegan.

Add a small amount of heavy cream or white wine to make the pesto creamier.

Add a dash of chili powder or red pepper flakes to make the pesto hotter.

Add some chopped mint, parsley, or basil for a more flavored pesto.

Add some chopped sun-dried tomatoes or crumbled bacon to the pesto for a unique spin.

RECIPE FOR BAKED SALMON WITH LEMON AND DILL

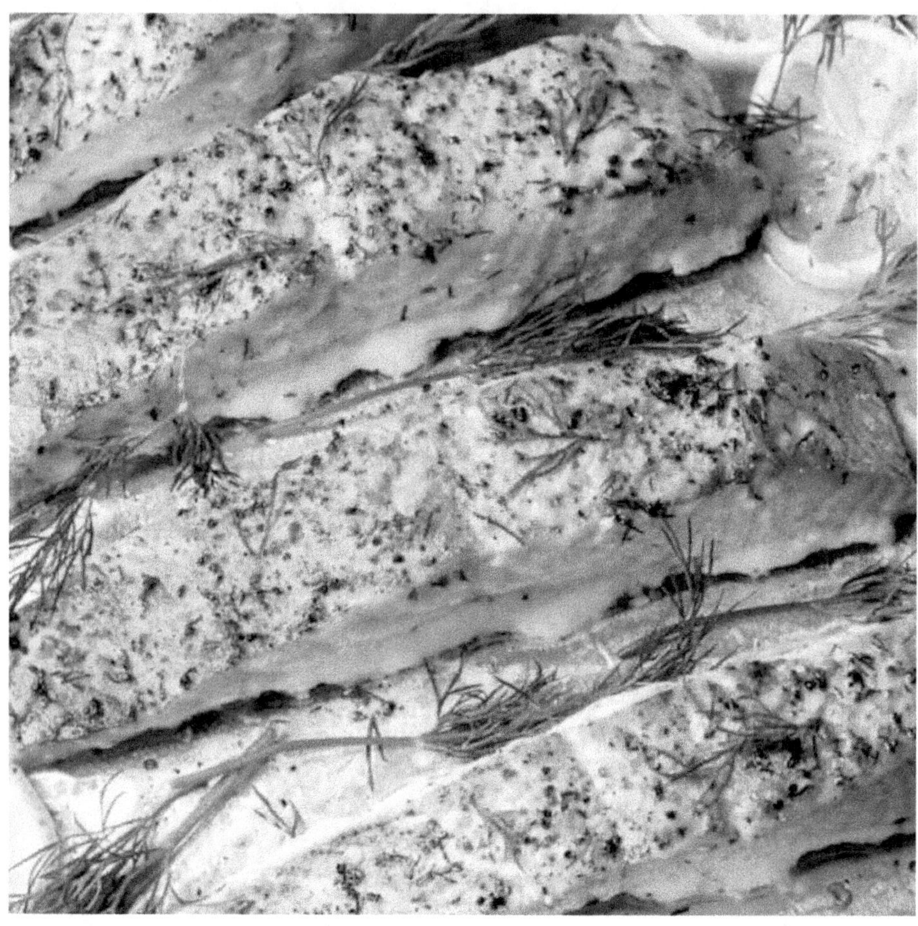

This recipe is tasty and nutritious, making it ideal for a midweek supper. It just needs a few ingredients and is simple to prepare. This is how you do it:

INGREDIENTS:

Four fillets of salmon (6–8 oz each)

Two tsp of olive oil

Two to three chopped garlic cloves; one finely sliced lemon

Two tablespoons of freshly chopped dill

To taste, add salt and black pepper.

slices of lemon as a garnish

Red onion slices cut thinly as a garnish are optional.

INSTRUCTIONS:

Warm up the oven:

- Turn the oven on to 375°F, or 190°C.

Get the salmon ready:

- Arrange the salmon fillets on a baking sheet that has been lightly oiled or covered with parchment paper.

Garnish the Salmon:

- Olive oil should be drizzled on the salmon fillets.
- Distribute evenly over the fillets the minced garlic, chopped dill, salt, and black pepper.

Cut up some lemons:

- Place slivers of lemon over each piece of salmon. For added taste, you can also tuck a lemon slice behind each fillet.

Salmon baked:

- Bake the salmon for 12 to 15 minutes per inch of thickness in a preheated oven, or until a fork can easily pierce it. The amount of time needed to cook depends on how thick your fillets are.

Finish:

- When the salmon is cooked, take it out of the oven and top it with more fresh dill and, if you like, thinly sliced red onion.

Advice:

The thickness of salmon fillets will determine how long to cook them. Generally, it takes 12 to 15 minutes for every inch of thickness, but it's crucial to test the fish's flakiness to ensure it's done.

Before baking, let the salmon sit for half an hour marinated in a mixture of olive oil, salt, pepper, lemon segments, and dill for maximum flavor.

Use parchment paper or lightly oil the baking pan to stop the salmon from sticking to it.

For the final one to two minutes, you can broil the salmon if you'd like a slightly crispier top but watch carefully to prevent overcooking.

In addition to being a tasty and low-carb alternative, this baked salmon with lemon and dill is also a nutritious choice. It's ideal for an easy and delicious supper.

NUTRITIONAL INFORMATION:

Size of serving: 1 fillet

300 calories

15g of fat

0g of carbohydrates

40g of protein

Modifications:

Add a little pinch of cayenne or red pepper flakes to the marinade for a hotter dish.

Add some minced shallots or garlic to the marinade for more flavor.

Before serving, top the salmon with a dollop of sour cream or yogurt for a creamier presentation.

Add some capers or olives to the marinade for a unique twist.

RECIPE FOR MEATBALLS AND SQUASH

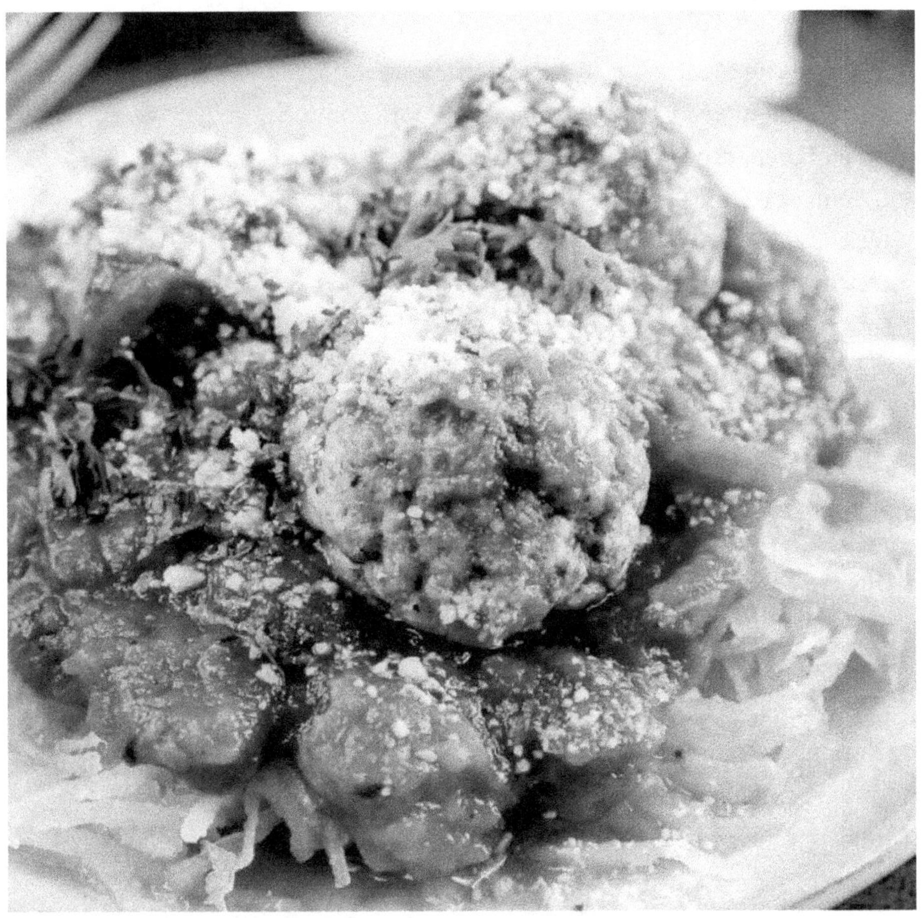

A tasty, filling low-carb substitute for regular pasta and meatballs is spaghetti squash and meatballs. This is how to prepare it:

INGREDIENTS:

For the squash spaghetti:
one spaghetti squash, medium
Olive oil.
Both black pepper and salt

Regarding the Meatballs:
One pound of ground beef (or beef and pork combined)
1/2 cup breadcrumbs (for a low-carb alternative, use almond meal)
1/4 cup of Parmesan cheese, grated
1/4 cup milk.
1/4 cup of freshly chopped parsley
One egg
one minced garlic clove
To taste, add salt and black pepper.

Regarding Sauce:
Two cups of tomato sauce (store-bought or homemade)
One tsp of dehydrated oregano
One tsp of dehydrated basil
To taste, add salt and black pepper.

Optional:
grated Parmigiano Reggiano
fresh parsley or basil, chopped

INSTRUCTIONS:

For the squash spaghetti:

- Turn the oven on to 375°F, or 190°C.
- Scoop off the seeds and strings after cutting the spaghetti squash in half lengthwise.
- After adding a little olive oil to each half, season with salt and black pepper.
- Spice up the squash
- Squash halves should be placed on a baking pan, and cut side down.
- Roast for 35 to 45 minutes in a preheated oven, or until the meat is fork-tender and readily scraped into "spaghetti" strands.
- Rub out the squash
- Scrape the cooked squash with a fork to form "spaghetti" strands. After putting the strands in a basin, set it aside.

Regarding the Meatballs:

- Ground beef, breadcrumbs (or almond meal), milk, chopped fresh parsley, minced garlic, egg, salt, and black pepper should all be combined in a mixing dish.
- Stir until all of the ingredients are incorporated.
- Create Meatballs:Shape the mixture into the size of meatballs that you want. Meatballs the size of a golf ball typically function well.
- Preheat the meatballs.Add a small amount of olive oil to a heated skillet over medium heat.
- The meatballs should be cooked for 15 to 20 minutes, or until they are browned on both sides.

Regarding Sauce:

- Heat the tomato sauce in a saucepan over medium heat.
- Add the salt, black pepper, dried basil, and dried oregano. For a few minutes, simmer.

Put Together the Dish

- Serve:Place the meatballs on top of the spaghetti squash after spooning the sauce over it.
- If preferred, garnish with chopped fresh parsley or basil and grated Parmesan cheese.

Advice:

To enhance the flavor of the sauce, you can add more ingredients such as red pepper flakes, sautéed onions, or garlic.

To suit your tastes, try experimenting with different ground meats or meatball seasonings.

Broil the scraped strands of spaghetti squash for a few minutes if you'd like a crispier texture.

With a healthy twist, spaghetti squash and meatballs offer the taste of a beloved classic dish in a low-carb, filling dish. Savor it as a healthy dinner choice.

NUTRITIONAL INFORMATION:

Size of serving: 1 dish
450 calories
20g of fat
30g of carbohydrates
40g of protein

Modifications:

Instead of using ground beef, try using ground turkey or ground chicken for a vegetarian twist on this recipe.

Use gluten-free bread crumbs to make this dish gluten-free.

Use low-fat or fat-free ground beef and reduced-fat or fat-free Parmesan cheese to make a healthier version of this recipe.

To enhance the taste of this recipe, incorporate chopped veggies like peppers, onions, and mushrooms into the meatballs.

Add some crumbled sausage or diced bacon to the meatballs for a unique flavor.

5

CHAPTER FOUR

SNACKS AND SIDES

RECIPE FOR ROASTED BRUSSEL SPROUTS WITH PARMESAN

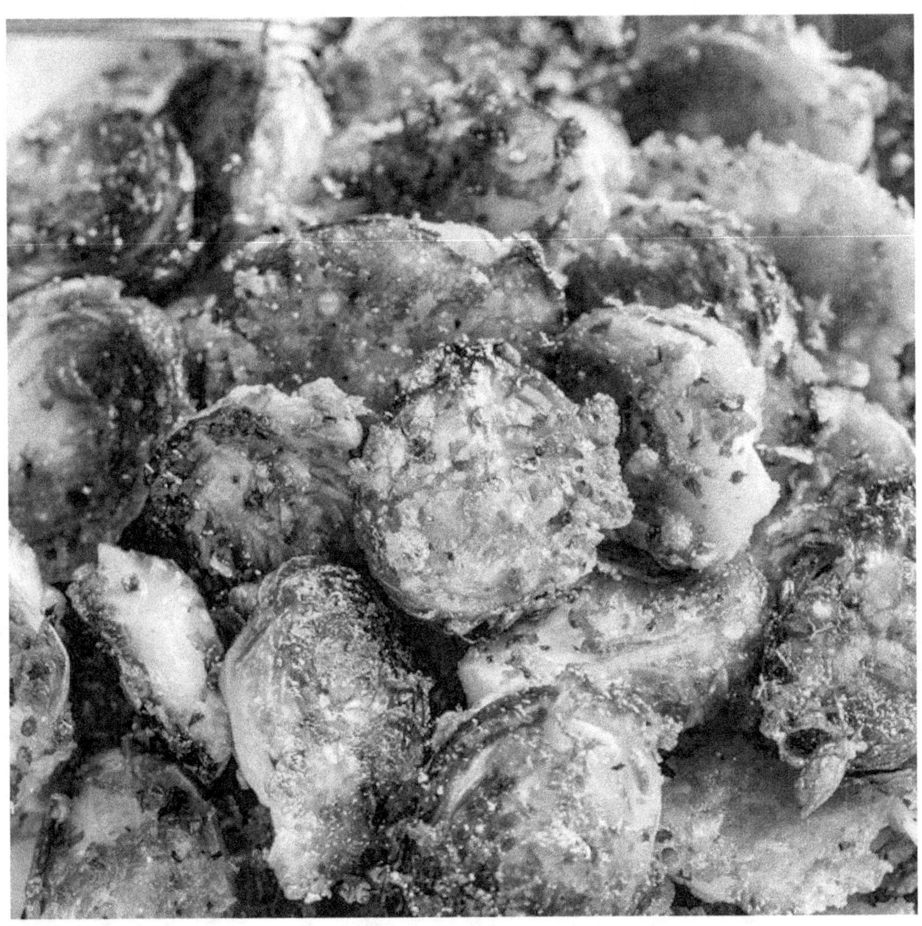

An easy and delicious side dish to make is roasted Brussels sprouts with Parmesan. This is how to prepare it:

INGREDIENTS:

One pound of halved and trimmed Brussels sprouts

Two to three tsp olive oil

To taste, add salt and black pepper.

1/4 cup of Parmesan cheese, grated

Crushed red pepper flakes are optional but add a little spiciness.

Fresh lemon juice is optional but adds a zesty touch.

INSTRUCTIONS:

- Warm up the oven:
- Set oven temperature to 400°F, or 200°C.
- Get the Brussels sprouts ready:Brussels sprouts should have their stem ends trimmed, and any yellowed or broken outer leaves should be removed.
- Halve every Brussels sprout.
- Toss with Olive Oil: Make sure the Brussels sprout halves are thoroughly covered by tossing them with olive oil in a sizable mixing dish.
- Toss the Brussels sprouts in a mixture of black pepper and salt. Add the crushed red pepper flakes now if you want your food spicy.
- Roast: Spread out the spiced Brussels sprouts in a single layer on a baking sheet.
- Roast for 20 to 25 minutes, or until they are soft and the edges are crispy, in a preheated oven. To ensure equal roasting, shake or stir the baking sheet a few times while it's cooking.
- Add Parmesan: During the final five minutes of roasting, cover the Brussels sprouts with grated Parmesan cheese. After the cheese has melted and become slightly crusty, put them back in the oven.
- Serve: Take the Parmesan-roasted Brussels sprouts out of the oven and place them on a platter. For an extra blast of citrus taste, you can optionally squeeze some fresh lemon juice over the top before serving.

Advice:

For even roasting, make sure the Brussels sprouts are arranged in a single layer on the oven sheet. If you crowd them, they may steam instead of roast.

Before roasting, sprinkle the Brussels sprouts with some garlic powder or balsamic vinegar for added flavor.

You are welcome to change the seasonings to suit your tastes. For added flavor, you can add more herbs or spices like garlic powder, thyme, or rosemary.

After washing and before tossing with olive oil, make sure the Brussels sprouts are thoroughly dry for a crispy texture.

The nutty flavor of Brussels sprouts and the rich, savory undertones of Parmesan cheese come together in a delicious side dish called roasted Brussels sprouts with Parmesan. It tastes great and added to any kind of food.

NUTRITIONAL INFORMATION:
portion size: one cup
120 calories
8g of fat
15g of carbohydrates
5g protein

Modifications:

Before roasting, sprinkle the Brussels sprouts with a small amount of cayenne pepper or red pepper flakes for a hotter dish.

Add some minced garlic or shallots to the Brussels sprouts before roasting them for an extra delicious entrée.

Before serving, top the Brussels sprouts with a dollop of sour cream or yogurt for a creamier meal.

Before roasting, sprinkle the Brussels sprouts with some chopped bacon or crumbled sausage for a unique flavor.

RECIPE FOR CUCUMBER AND CREAM CHEESE ROLL-UPS

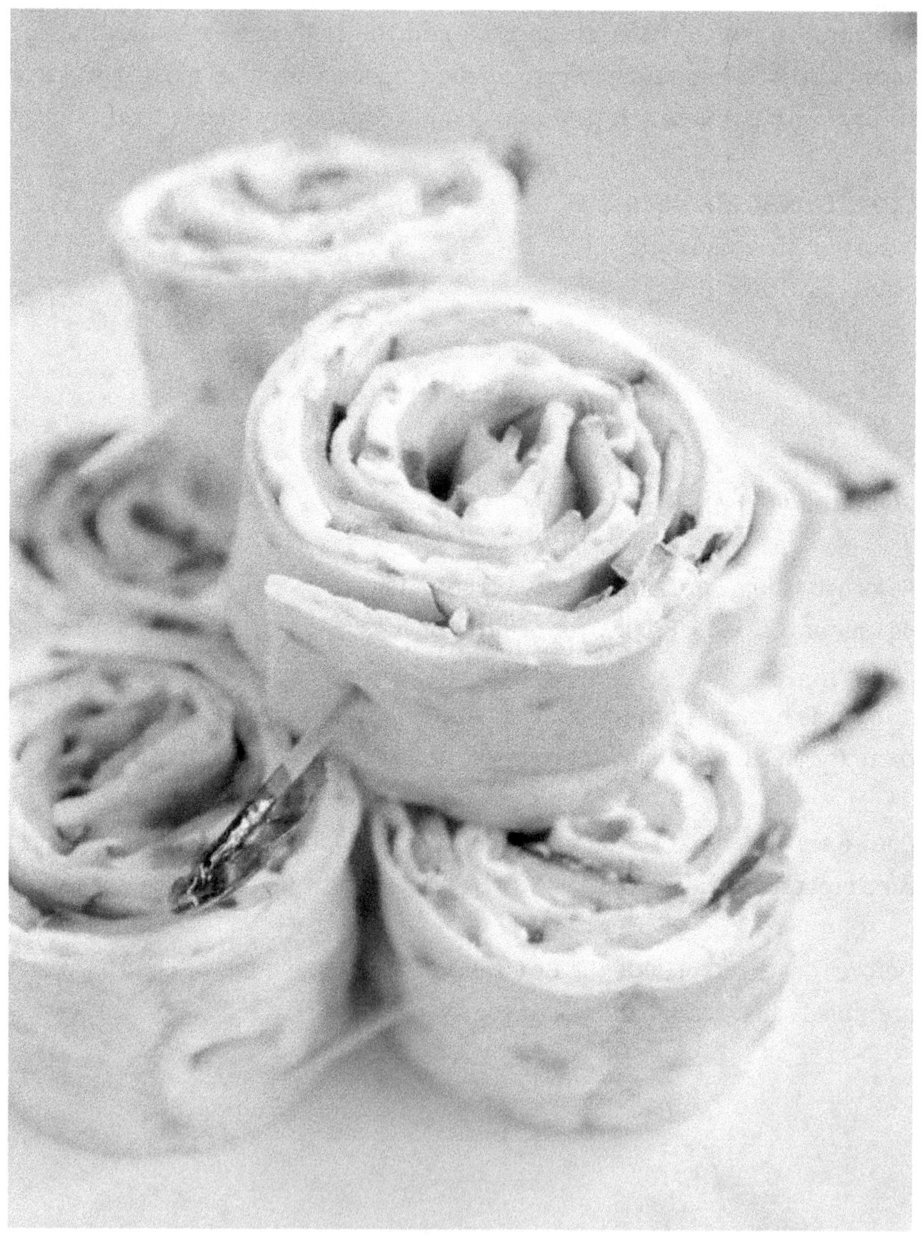

Low-carb appetizers or snacks like cucumber and cream cheese roll-ups are easy and pleasant. This is how to prepare them:

INGREDIENTS:

1 big cucumber

Four ounces, or half a cup, softened cream cheese

One tablespoon of freshly chopped chives and two tablespoons of freshly chopped dill

To taste, add salt and black pepper.

Prosciutto or smoked salmon is optional

INSTRUCTIONS:

- Get the cucumber ready:
- If desired, peel the cucumber after giving it a good wash. You can leave some skin on for color and texture to create a visually appealing presentation.
- Cut the cucumber in half
- Peel and slice the cucumber lengthwise into long, thin strips using a vegetable peeler or mandoline slicer.

Get the cream cheese mixture ready.

- Put the softened cream cheese, finely chopped fresh dill, finely chopped fresh chives, and a dash of black pepper and salt in a mixing dish.
- Blend until every component is thoroughly combined.
- Lay out one cucumber strip at a time to assemble the roll-ups.
- Each cucumber strip should have a thin layer of the cream cheese mixture running the length of it.
- Place a thin slice of prosciutto or smoked salmon on top of the cream cheese layer, if desired.
- Roll Up the Cucumbers: Starting at one end of the cucumber strip, carefully roll it toward the other.

• If necessary, fasten with a toothpick.

To firm up and intensify the flavors, refrigerate the cucumber and cream cheese roll-ups for 15 to 30 minutes.

Provide:
Place the roll-ups onto a dish for serving.
Garnish with extra dill, chives, or a dash of black pepper, if desired.

Advice:
Feel free to adjust the amount of each herb and spice in the cream cheese mixture to your personal preference. For added taste, try adding a dash of lemon juice or a teaspoon of garlic powder.

Spread the full-fat cream cheese mixture over the cucumber slices after beating it until it becomes smooth.

You may customize these roll-ups a lot. Other fillings like roast beef, smoked turkey, or your preferred cheese can be used.

For those seeking a low-carb alternative, cucumber and cream cheese roll-ups are a refreshing, crisp, and creamy snack or appetizer. They are a fun and welcome addition to any get-together.

NUTRITIONAL INFORMATION:
Size of serving: one roll-up
50 calories
Fat (3g)
5g of carbohydrates
2g protein

Variations:
To make each cucumber roll-up a more substantial snack, tuck a slice of

ham or smoked salmon inside.

For an alternative flavor profile, try goat or feta cheese instead of cream cheese.

For a gluten-free version, try using whole-wheat tortillas in place of the cucumber slices.

For added taste and nutrition, cut some veggies, like tomatoes, onions, or bell peppers, and add them to the cream cheese mixture.

Arrange the cucumber roll-ups with other starters like cheese and crackers, bruschetta, or shrimp cocktail on a tray.

AVOCADO WITH VEGETABLE STICKS

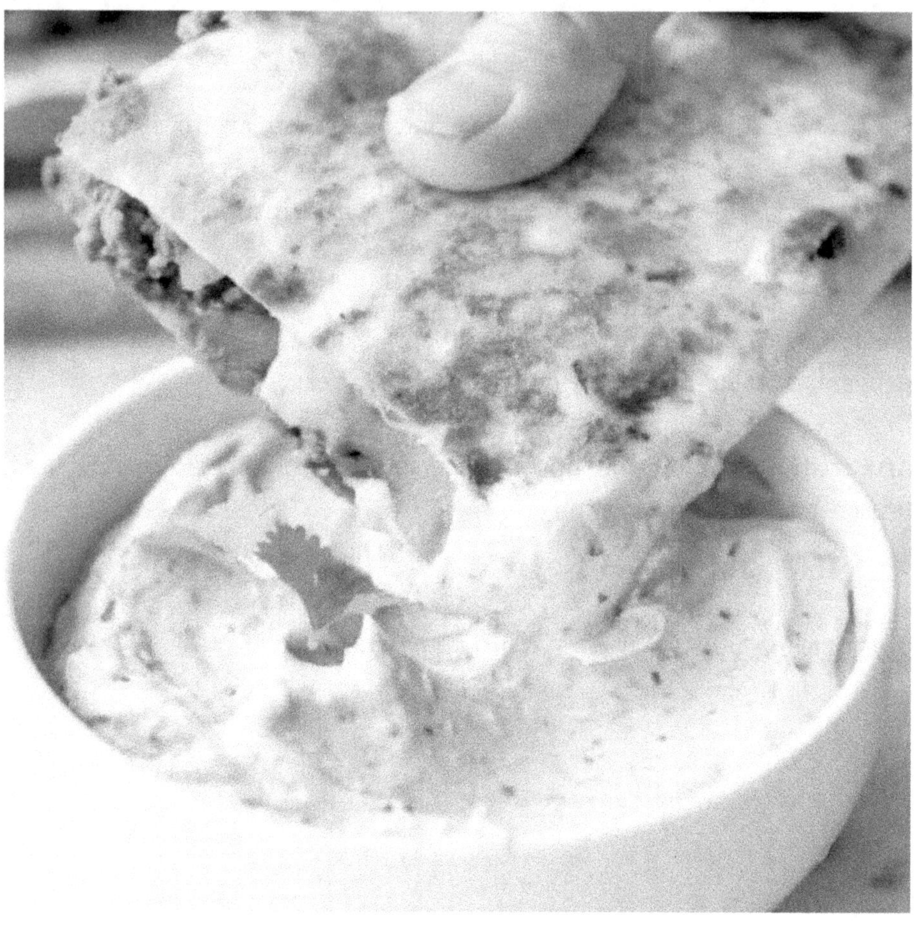

A tasty and nutritious dip that goes well with vegetable sticks is guacamole. It is a delicious and nutritious way to get your recommended daily intake of vegetables. You may learn how to prepare guacamole and what vegetables go well with it by following this recipe.

Ingredients

two ripe avocados

One little red onion, chopped finely

one or two minced garlic cloves

One or two tomatoes, chopped;

one lime;

one-fourth cup of freshly chopped cilantro

To taste, add salt and black pepper.

Optional: finely sliced 1-2 jalapeño peppers for added spiciness

Carrot Sticks:

Select a range of vibrant vegetables, including cherry tomatoes, bell peppers, cucumbers, and celery. They should be cleaned, peeled, and sliced or sticks for dipping.

INSTRUCTIONS:

The guacamole ready:

- Remove the pits from the avocados, cut them in half, and scoop the flesh into a mixing bowl.
- Using a fork or potato masher, mash the avocados until they are as smooth as you wish (some people like their avocados chunky, while others love it smooth).
- Add Ingredients: Finely diced red onion, minced garlic, diced tomatoes, lime juice, and chopped cilantro should all be added to the mashed avocados.
- Add finely diced jalapeño peppers if desired heat.
- To taste, add salt and black pepper for seasoning. Start with a modest quantity and change it to suit your tastes.
- Mix and Taste: Using a whisk, thoroughly mix each item until thoroughly incorporated.

If necessary, taste the guacamole and add extra lime juice, salt, or pepper to balance the spices.

Get the veggie sticks ready:

- Clean, peel, and slice or stick the colored vegetables of your choice.

· Serve: Arrange the vegetable sticks for dipping around the guacamole in a serving basin.

Advice:

To add even more flavor to your guacamole, try adding extra cilantro, a splash of spicy sauce, or a touch of cumin.

If you are not serving the guacamole right away, save the avocado pits and add them to the mixture to help keep it from browning.

Use a food processor or blender to make your guacamole smoother if that's your preference.

Vegetable sticks and guacamole make a filling and healthy snack or appetizer. The fresh, crisp vegetables make a delicious pairing with the creamy guacamole. Have fun!

NUTRITIONAL INFORMATION:

Serving size: 1 cup of vegetable sticks and 1/4 cup of guacamole

150 calories

12g of fat

10g of carbohydrates

3g protein

Modifications:

To add more taste and nutrients to the guacamole, cut an onion or tomato.

For a more substantial dip, mix in some cooked black beans or corn with the guacamole.

Serve the guacamole as a traditional Mexican appetizer, with tortilla chips in place of veggie sticks.

For extra richness, top the guacamole with a dollop of yogurt or sour cream.

For a taste and color boost, add some fresh parsley or cilantro to the guacamole.

6

CHAPTER FIVE

BUDGET-FRIENDLY DESSERTS

RECIPE FOR CHOCOLATE AVOCADO MOUSSE

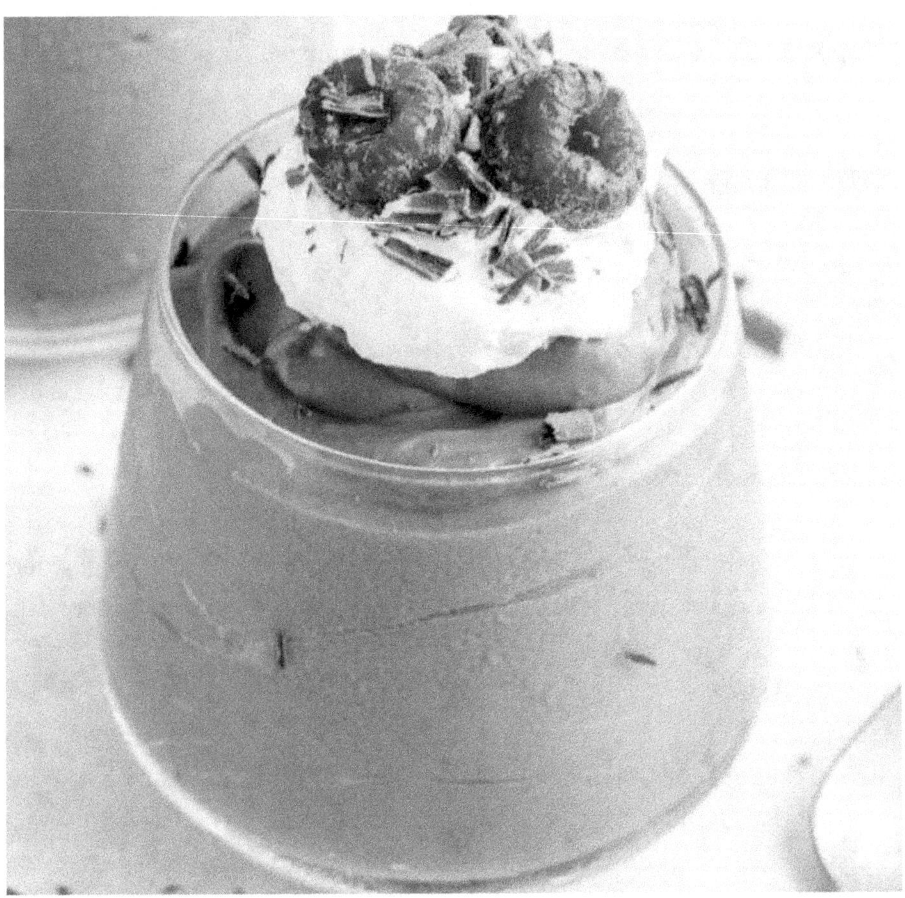

A tasty and healthy substitute for classic chocolate mousse is chocolate avocado mousse. It's quite satisfying, creamy, and rich. This is how to prepare it:

INGREDIENTS:

Two plump avocados

1/4 cup chocolate powder, unsweetened

1/4 cup maple syrup or honey, adjusted to taste

1/4 cup milk, either non-dairy or dairy

One tsp vanilla essence

Add a dash of salt

Toppers: grated chocolate, fresh berries, or whipped cream are optional.

INSTRUCTIONS:

Get the avocados ready:

- Halve the avocados, remove the pits, and transfer the flesh to a food processor or blender.

Mix the Concoction:

- To the blender or food processor, add the unsweetened cocoa powder, milk, vanilla extract, honey (or maple syrup), and a small amount of salt.

Puree until silky:

- Mix the ingredients in a blender until the mixture is creamy and fully smooth. To make sure everything is well blended, you might need to pause and scrape down the sides several times.

Smell and Modify:

- Once you taste the mousse, you can modify the sweetness to suit your tastes. If desired, add extra honey or maple syrup.

Optional:

- Before serving, place the mousse in the fridge for at least 30 minutes if you would like it cold.

Provide:
Spoon into serving dishes the chocolate avocado mousse into.

For extra taste and texture, you can choose to top with whipped cream, fresh berries, or grated chocolate.

Advice:

Use nondairy milk, such as coconut or almond milk, for a vegan or dairy-free variation.

Try a variety of sweeteners to see which works best for your diet or taste preferences. Agave syrup, stevia, or even mashed bananas can be used.

Although the mousse keeps well in the fridge for a day or two, serving it fresh is recommended.

Rich and creamy, chocolate avocado mousse is a dessert that is loaded with antioxidants and good fats. It's ideal for sating your want for chocolate without feeling guilty. Savor this tasty treat!

NUTRITIONAL INFORMATION:
   Portion size: half a cup
   250 calories
   18g of fat
   20g of carbohydrates
   5g protein

Modifications:

Add 1 tablespoon of instant coffee powder to the food processor with the remaining ingredients to make a mousse with a coffee taste.

Add one teaspoon of mint extract to the food processor with the remaining ingredients to make a mousse with a mint taste.

To make a mousse with a peanut butter taste, combine the remaining ingredients in a food processor with 1/4 cup of natural peanut butter.

Once the mousse has been made, whisk in 1/4 cup small chocolate chips to make a chocolate chip mousse.

Add a scoop of your preferred ice cream and a drizzle of chocolate sauce to the mousse for a unique twist.

RECIPE FOR BERRY CHIA SEED PUDDING

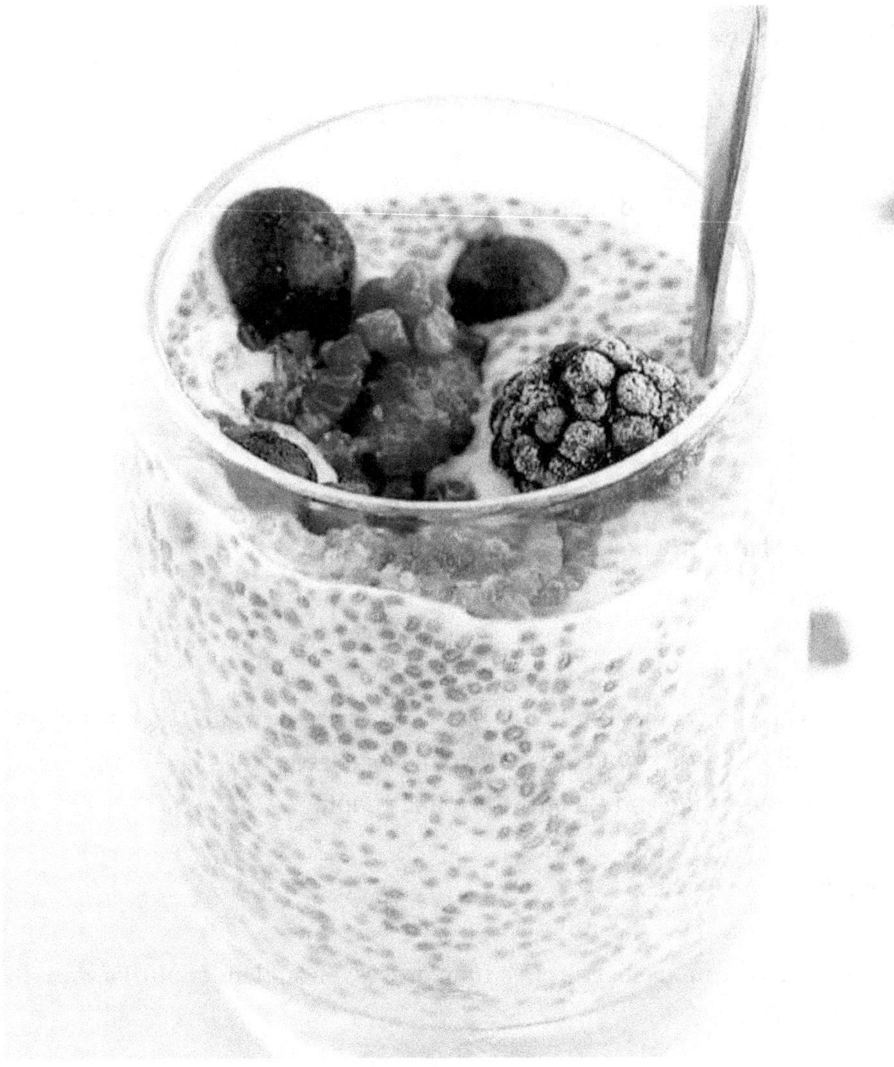

A tasty and nutritious treat that can be eaten for breakfast or as a healthful dessert is berry chia seed pudding. This is how to prepare it:

INGREDIENTS:

- Half a cup of chia seeds
- One cup of milk (almond or coconut milk, or dairy or non-dairy)

- 1–2 teaspoons of maple syrup or honey, adjusted to taste
- One-half tsp vanilla extract
- One cup of mixed berries, including raspberries, blueberries, and straw-berries
- Extra berries, sliced almonds, or a honey drizzle are optional garnishes.

INSTRUCTIONS:

Get the Chia Seed Mixture Ready:

- Chia seeds, milk, honey (or maple syrup), and vanilla essence should all be combined in a bowl. Mix thoroughly to blend.

Give It A Go:

- Chia seed mixture should be chilled for at least two to three hours, or overnight if the bowl is covered. The chia seeds will soak up the liquid during this time and become thick like pudding.

Combinate the Berries:

- Process the mixed berries in a food processor or blender until a smooth purée forms.

Put the Pudding Together:

- Remove the combination of chia seeds from the refrigerator.
- Layer the berry puree and the chia seed pudding into serving dishes or glasses. You can either pour the berry puree on top or alternate the layers to produce a marbled appearance.

Optional:

- To allow the flavors to mingle, put the assembled pudding back in the fridge for around half an hour.

Provide:

Garnish with more berries, sliced almonds, or a drizzle of honey just before serving.

Advice:

You can experiment with different amounts of honey or maple syrup to get the desired sweetness.

Blend the berries until they are pureed before adding them to the bowl for a smoother pudding.

You may add richness and extra creaminess to your chia seed pudding by using Greek yogurt or full-fat coconut milk.

You are welcome to add your preferred fruits, nuts, or seeds as toppings.

Delicious and adaptable, berry chia seed pudding can be made to suit your preferences. It's a wonderful way to make use of the health advantages of chia seeds and the inherent sweetness of berries. It's a lovely delicacy for breakfast or dessert.

NUTRITIONAL INFORMATION:

portion size: one cup

200 calories

10g of fat

25g of carbohydrates

5g protein

Modifications:

Use coconut milk, pineapple, and mango in the pudding for a touch of the tropics.

Add one tablespoon of unsweetened cocoa powder to the pudding recipe for a chocolaty touch.

Add 1/4 cup of natural peanut butter to the pudding recipe for a peanut butter twist.

Add 1/4 cup pureed pumpkin, 1/2 teaspoon cinnamon, and 1/4 teaspoon nutmeg to the pudding mixture to make it taste like pumpkin pie.

Before adding the pudding, create a layer at the bottom of the jar with yogurt, granola, or fresh fruit for a creative variation.

RECIPE FOR KETO-FRIENDLY PEANUT BUTTER COOKIES

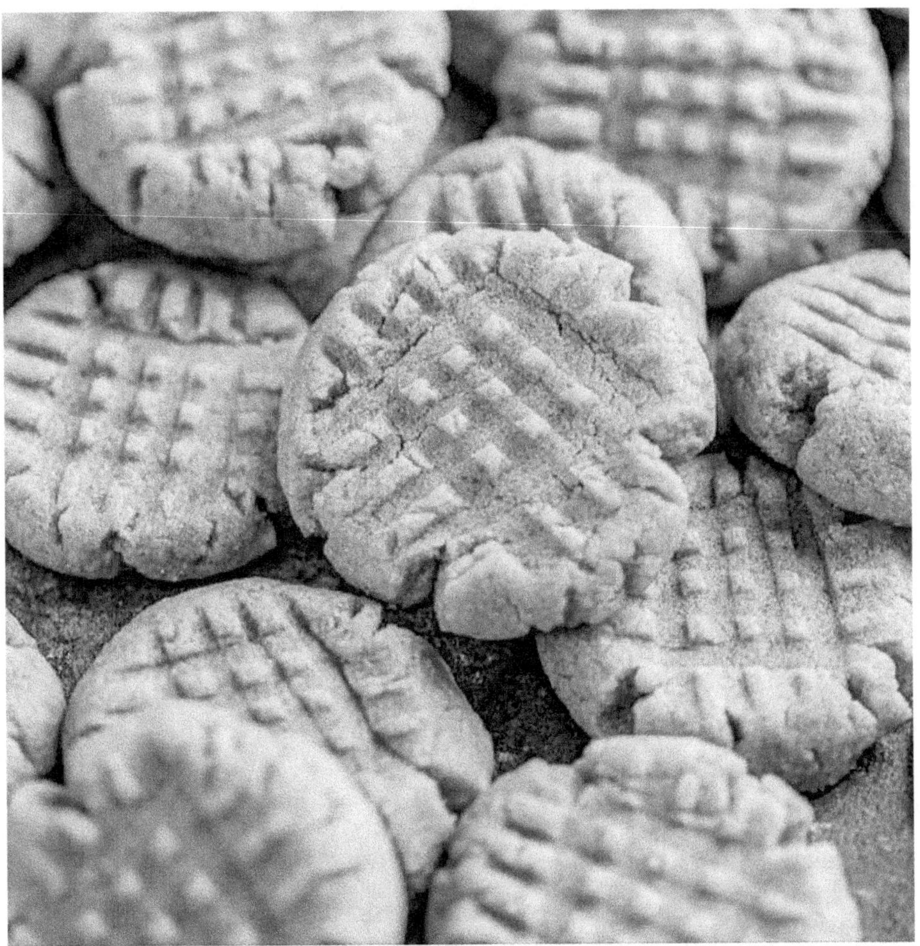

Peanut butter cookies that are keto-friendly are a tasty low-carb treat. This is a basic recipe for making delicious cookies.

INGREDIENTS:

One cup of natural, unsweetened peanut butter

Half a cup of erythritol, or any other sugar that is keto-friendly

One big egg

One tsp vanilla essence

One-half tsp baking soda

A scant pinch of salt.

INSTRUCTIONS:

Warm up the oven:

- Set the oven temperature to 350°F (175°C).

Get the dough ready:

- The natural peanut butter, egg, baking soda, vanilla extract, granulated erythritol (or your preferred keto-friendly sweetener), and a dash of salt should all be combined in a mixing dish.

Mix the Substances:

- Mix the ingredients until a nice dough for cookies forms. It should be simple to deal with; you can mix it with a spoon or your hands.

Form the Biscuits:

- Roll out pieces of dough to make 1-inch (2.5 cm) balls. Transfer these balls to a baking sheet covered with parchment paper.

Press the Cookies Flat:

- Each cookie should be flattened using a fork to make a crosshatch design. To keep the fork from sticking, dip it into the water in between pressing.

Cook:

- For ten to twelve minutes, bake the cookies in a preheated oven. Their core should remain soft and the margins should be just a hint of gold.

After a few minutes of cooling on the baking sheet, move the cookies to a wire rack to finish cooling.

Provide:

The cookies are ready to be enjoyed as a keto-friendly treat once they have cooled.

Advice:

Make sure the peanut butter you use is natural and free of additional sugars. For variation, you can also use different nut butter, including almond butter.

You can add more or less sweetener to suit your preferred level of sweetness.

When these cookies are first made, they can be very fragile, so handle them carefully until they cool and harden.

For people on a ketogenic diet or trying to cut back on sugar, these delicious low-carb peanut butter cookies make a great snack or dessert. Savor their flavorful peanut butter without feeling guilty!

NUTRITIONAL INFORMATION:

Size of serving: one cookie

150 calories

12g of fat

2g of carbohydrates

5g protein

Modifications:

You can add 1/4 cup of unsweetened cocoa powder to the batter to make chocolate peanut butter cookies.

Place your preferred keto-friendly jam between the cookies to make a peanut butter and jelly sandwich.

Add 1/4 cup of small chocolate chips to the batter to make a peanut butter and chocolate chip cookie.

Add 1/4 cup of shredded coconut to the batter and stir to make a peanut butter and coconut cookie.

Drizzle some melted peanut butter or chocolate sauce over the cookies for a unique twist.

7

CHAPTER SIX

MEAL PLANNING AND SHOPPING TIPS

Careful planning and economical item selection are necessary to create a low-carb, budget-friendly meal plan that maintains a healthy, balanced diet. Here's a step-by-step tutorial to get you going:

Step 1: Establish a Budget

Establish a weekly or monthly grocery spending limit. This will direct your selection of ingredients and meal planning.

Step 2: Make a meal plan

Determine the number of meals and snacks you will require each week. This usually covers breakfast, lunch, dinner, and a couple of snacks.

Step 3: Select Foods Low in Carbs

Find low-carbohydrate foods that you can afford. Low-cost and low-carb staples include eggs, canned tuna, chicken thighs, tofu, cauliflower, zucchini, and cabbage.

Step 4: Examine Recipes with Low Carbs

Look in cookbooks or online for reasonably priced low-carb dishes. Make use of social media, blogs, and websites to get ideas and inspiration for your meal plan.

Step 5: Purchase in bulk

To save money, buy non-perishable low-carb foods in bulk. This comprises seeds, nuts, and tinned fish as well as vegetables.

Step 6: Vegetables in Season

Seasonal low-carb fruits and veggies are a better choice because they are usually less expensive. For discounts, visit your local farmers' market.

Step 7: Make a weekly meal plan

Make a weekly meal plan with low-carb dishes. To reduce waste, make sure you use similar foods in each meal.

Step 8: Batch-Cooking

Think about cooking in bulk on the weekends. Throughout the week, this can help save time and money. Make a lot of protein and low-carb side dishes.

Step 9: Store and Freeze

To avoid food waste, store food in sealed containers and freeze additional portions.

Step 10: Observe Your Spending

As you prepare meals and go grocery shopping, keep an eye on your expenditures. If needed, modify your meal plan to keep within your means.

Making a low-carb, cost-effective meal plan involves some advanced preparation and structuring. You may have tasty, nourishing meals without going over budget by using inexpensive, low-carb foods and reducing food waste.

An example of a low-carb, economical meal plan is:

Day One:

Eggs scrambled with spinach and feta for breakfast.

Tuna salad lettuce wraps for lunch.

Dinner is broccoli and baked chicken thighs.

Day Two:

Greek yogurt parfait with berries for breakfast.

Lunch is a breakfast wrap with avocado and bacon.

Soup with cauliflower and broccoli for dinner.

Day Three:

Celery sticks with peanut butter for breakfast.

Pesto-crusted zucchini noodles for lunch.

Dinner is fish baked with dill and lemon.

Day Four:

Chia seed pudding and almond milk for breakfast.

Meatballs and spaghetti squash for lunch.

Dinner is Parmesan-crusted roasted Brussels sprouts.

Day Five

Breakfast: Previous recipe's low-carb peanut butter cookies.

Guacamole and vegetable sticks for lunch.

Dinner is chia seed pudding with berries (a low-carb treat).

Cost-effective Atkins Diet Shopping Techniques

Budget-conscious Atkins Diet shopping will help you avoid going overboard and keep you on track. *The following are some tips to help you stick to the diet and save money:*

Arrange Your Food: Arrange your meals for the week ahead of time to prevent impulsive and possibly expensive food decisions.

Establish a shopping list:Make a thorough shopping list according to your food plan. Follow the list to prevent purchasing extraneous things.

Buy Large: To save money, buy low-carb, non-perishable goods in bulk, such as canned veggies, nuts, and seeds.

Seek out discounts and sales: Look for discounts, coupons, and retail flyers. Purchase things that are promoted or on sale to save money.

Visit discount retailers: When purchasing low-carb essentials like spices, tuna in cans, and olive oil, think about going to bulk or discount stores.

Invest in canned and frozen foods: Low-carb canned and frozen veggies and protein sources can be less expensive than fresh. They last longer on the shelf as well.

Acquire Generic Names: Rather than name brands, choose generic or store-brand goods. They are frequently just as good but less costly.

Steer clear of pre-packaged low-carb items: Low-carb prepared dishes might be expensive. Rather, purchase complete supplies and make dishes from scratch.

Apply Remainders:Make leftovers a part of your meal plans to cut down on food waste and save costs.

Select Less Expensive Protein Sources: Compared to expensive cuts of meat, eggs, chicken thighs, ground beef, and tofu are frequently more affordable options.

Select Seasonal Vegetables: Seasonally available, low-carb fruits and veggies are usually more reasonably priced.

Limit Specialty Items and Snacks: Specialty low-carb foods and snacks might be pricey. Treat them just sometimes.

Purchase in Smaller Amounts: To reduce waste, only buy as much fresh produce as you would eat. This might be more economical.

Employ Reward Systems: Utilize store loyalty programs to receive rebates or discounts on your purchases.

Examine Costs: To find the best deal for your money, compare costs per unit (such as price per ounce or gram).

Cook in Groups: To cut back on takeaway or eating out, prepare larger portions of meals and freeze them for later use.

Pay Attention to Expiration Dates:you prevent food waste, make sure you use products with shorter expiration dates first.

Minimize Dining Out: Spending less on takeout and restaurants can result in large financial savings. Make your own Atkins-approved meals instead.

Sign up for a Warehouse Club: When buying low-carb products in bulk, warehouse clubs can save you money. If purchasing a subscription makes sense for you financially, do so.

Remain Updated: Keep yourself informed on affordable, Atkins-compliant low-carb recipes and meal planning tips.

You can control your grocery costs and follow a low-carb Atkins diet by using these tactics. Budget-friendly purchasing and careful planning can be achieved without sacrificing your nutritional objectives.

8

CHAPTER SEVEN

Budget-Friendly Ingredient Swaps

You can stretch the budget of your dishes by substituting ingredients. To cut costs, try these popular ingredient substitutions:

To make cornstarch, flour:

Instead of using cornstarch as a thickening agent, use all-purpose flour. It's a more affordable option.

Nuts with Oats:

Oats can be used in place of nuts in recipes that call for them to achieve a comparable texture at a reduced cost.

For Sour Cream, Use Greek Yogurt:

Sour cream can be swapped out for Greek yogurt in recipes for a more affordable, high-protein option.

Swap Fresh Tomatoes with Canned Tomatoes:

In soups, stews, and sauces, canned tomatoes—especially when they're on sale—replace fresh tomatoes at a lower cost.

Oats rolled into crumbs for bread:

When ground, rolled oats can be used in place of bread crumbs in recipes, providing a healthier and less expensive alternative.

Ground Beef with Ground Turkey:

Ground turkey can be substituted for ground beef in a variety of recipes and is frequently less expensive than ground beef.

For chicken breasts, use chicken thighs:

When compared to chicken breasts, chicken thighs are usually more flavorful and more affordable.

Fresh vs. Frozen Vegetables:

In many recipes, frozen vegetables might be a more affordable option than fresh ones.

Rice with Pasta:

When compared to rice, pasta is frequently less expensive and can be used in similar recipes like casseroles or stir-fries.

Swap Canned Beans with Dried Beans:

When weighed against canned beans, dried beans are a more affordable choice. For recipes, soak and cook them as needed.

For chicken pieces, the entire chicken:

Generally speaking, a complete chicken costs less per pound than individual parts. It's easy to cut into pieces by yourself.

Ground Pork for Sausage on the Ground:

If a recipe calls for ground sausage, you might be able to save money by substituting ground pork with your favorite seasonings.

For Ground Meat, Use Lentils:

In recipes like spaghetti sauce or chili, lentils can partially or completely substitute the ground beef, cutting expenses and increasing fiber content.

Beef or Chicken Stock with Vegetable Broth:

For vegans in particular, vegetable broth can frequently be used in place of chicken or beef broth in recipes.

For vinegar, use lemon juice:

In many recipes, lemon juice can be used in place of vinegar to add a cheap, fresh acidic element.

Bananas Mashed for Eggs:

Mashed ripe bananas can save money and add natural sweetness to baked goods by substituting for eggs.

Vinegar with Milk for Buttermilk:

For recipes that call for buttermilk, mix vinegar and milk to make a replacement.

Replace Ricotta Cheese with Cottage Cheese:

In lasagnas and other recipes, cottage cheese can be used in place of ricotta cheese at a lower cost.

Heat-Related Butter:

For a less expensive option, you can use cooking oil for butter in several recipes.

Sugar and Cinnamon for Vanilla Extract:

In certain recipes, you can substitute sugar and cinnamon for vanilla extract for a less expensive choice.

You may create tasty and economical dinners while controlling your grocery budget by substituting these ingredients. Make sure to modify the substitutions according to your dietary restrictions as well as the particular specifications of your recipes.

How to Maximize Remaining Food

Utilizing leftovers to their full potential is a frugal and astute method of cutting down on food wastage and saving time in the kitchen. The following advice will help you maximize the use of your leftovers:

Meal Planning: Keep leftovers in mind when making your meal plans. If you're having roasted chicken for supper, think about what you could make with the leftovers the following day.

Appropriate Storage: Quickly refrigerate leftovers in sealed containers. Put the dates on containers so you can monitor their freshness.

Reimagine Recipes: Use leftovers in inventive ways. Use leftover rice for fried rice, or use the roasted vegetables from yesterday night to make a frittata.

Soups and Stews: You can make soups and stews with leftover meats and vegetables. Just add the broth and season to taste.

Casseroles: To make casseroles, mix different leftovers with cheese, sauce, and a topping such as mashed potatoes or bread crumbs.

Salads: For a quick and nutritious lunch, top a fresh salad with leftover proteins, such as chicken, beef, or fish.

Omelets and Quiches: For a hearty breakfast or brunch, leftover meats, cheeses, and veggies can be put into omelets and quiches.

Sandwiches and Wraps: For a fast lunch, make sandwiches or wraps with leftover meats, grilled vegetables, and condiments.

Freeze for Later: Freeze leftovers for later use if you can't finish them immediately away. Casseroles, stews, and soups freeze nicely.

Make Your Own Broth: To make your own homemade broth, save the leftover vegetables and animal bones. It is economical and improves the taste of food.

Pasta dishes: To make a quick and easy dinner, combine cooked pasta with leftover proteins, veggies, and sauces.

Stir-Fries: For a delicious, low-cost meal, stir-fry leftover veggies and proteins with soy sauce.

Snack Plates: For an easy and filling snack, assemble leftover cheeses, meats, fruits, and vegetables into snack plates.

Label and Date: Make sure to mark leftovers with the day they were made and eat older leftovers before fresh ones.

Keep Safety in Mind: Be mindful of food safety. To prevent spoiling, leftovers should be eaten within a fair amount of time.

Give to Others: If you have more leftovers than you can eat, give them to your neighbors, relatives, or friends.

Learn how to cook with no waste by utilizing every component of your ingredients. Use citrus peels, for instance, to make homemade stock or zest.

Every week, set aside a "leftover night" to clean out the refrigerator and avoid wasting any food.

To ensure that you don't forget about your leftovers in the back of the refrigerator, make an inventory note of them.

Cooking in Bulk: Arrange to prepare large amounts of foods such as lasagna or chili, which may be frozen and portioned for later use.

Utilizing leftovers to their full potential not only saves you money but also lessens food waste, which benefits both the environment and your pocketbook. Having ready-made meals available might also help you save time on hectic days.

9

CONCLUSION

With careful planning and cost-effective decisions, it is totally feasible to succeed on the Atkins Diet without going bankrupt. The following advice will help you stick to the Atkins Diet on a tight budget:

Arrange Your Food: Make a weekly meal plan that follows the guidelines of the Atkins Diet. You'll shop more effectively and waste less food if you do this.

Buy Large: To save money, buy low-carb pantry essentials in bulk, such as nuts, seeds, and canned veggies.

Seasonal Vegetables: Select seasonal, lower-carb fruits and veggies; these are frequently fresher and more reasonably priced.

Cut Back on Pre-Packaged Foods: Steer clear of pricey, pre-packaged low-carb items. Rather, choose complete foods and make your meals yourself.

Protein Sources at a Low Cost: Choose affordable protein sources such ground beef, eggs, and chicken thighs.

Fresh vs. Frozen: Think for frozen berries and veggies that are low in carbs;

they might be more affordable and have a longer shelf life than fresh.

Retailer Brands: Store-brand or generic products are often more affordable while maintaining a comparable level of quality to major brands.

Prepare Meals and Cook in Bulk: Cook in large quantities and freeze individual servings. This reduces the necessity of going out to eat or getting takeout on hectic days.

Easy Recipes: Stay with easy dishes that are easier to prepare and use less ingredients.

Crafty Snacks: Create your own low-carb snacks, such as cheese crisps, vegetable chips, or homemade beef jerky.

Remaining Magic: Use leftovers in inventive ways. Make dinner from last night something intriguing and new.

Select Low-Cost Fats: Make use of affordable, healthful fat sources like avocados, butter, and vegetable oils.

Value Superior to Quantity: Put quality first when selecting low-carb foods, even if it means making fewer purchases. Nutrient-dense, high-quality foods may be more filling, allowing you to eat less in general.

Meal Prep Dishes: To portion out meals and cut down on waste, get some reusable meal prep containers.

Ice-Cold Berries: When making smoothies and dishes that call for fresh berries, use frozen berries. They're accessible all year round and frequently cost less.

Keep Convenience Items Away: Avoid low-carb convenience foods like bars and smoothies that are already made. Generally speaking, they cost more than complete foods.

Discounts and Sales: For low-carb ingredients, keep an eye out for coupons, deals, and discounts.

Waste-Free Cooking:Use every portion of the ingredient when cooking to reduce waste. For example, make homemade stock from vegetable leftovers.

Divide the Work: Think about buying ingredients in bulk and splitting the cost if you have friends or family who are on the Atkins Diet.

Web-Based Resources: Making the most of inexpensive products, careful preparation, and straightforward cooking are all necessary to succeed on the Atkins Diet without going over budget. You can successfully adhere to the Atkins Diet and stick to your budget by using these techniques.

Your Path to Atkins Living on a Budget

Setting out on a quest for affordable Living the Atkins lifestyle is enjoyable and doable. Here is a roadmap to assist you successfully traverse this path:

Make definite goals:

   Establish your spending limit and your goals for the Atkins Diet. The first step is to recognize your financial boundaries.

Arrange Your Food:

   Make a weekly meal plan that includes your snacks, dinner, lunch, and morning. Adhere to your strategy to reduce food waste.

Buy Wisely:

   When feasible, buy low-carb basics in bulk. To save money, stick to store-brand and seasonal products.

Put Protein First:

Invest in reasonably priced sources of protein, such as ground beef, eggs, and chicken thighs. These are reasonably priced and provide decent nourishment.

Reduce the Use of Pre-Packaged Goods:

Steer clear of pricey prepackaged low-carb items. Choose foods that are whole, fresh, or barely processed.

Select canned or frozen food.

Berries, canned products, and frozen low-carb veggies can be more affordable and have a longer shelf life.

Easy Cooking:

Put an emphasis on easy homemade dishes that may be made faster and with less ingredients.

Meal Planning

Meal preparation and batch cooking are cost- and time-effective. Make more food and store any leftovers in the freezer.

Make Creative Use of Leftovers:

Use leftovers in creative ways. Make a fresh, exciting dinner out of yesterday's leftovers.

Value Superior to Quantity:

Put a higher priority on nutrient-dense, premium ingredients, even if it means purchasing them in lower amounts. You'll eat less overall and feel fuller.

Crafty Snacks:

Make your own jerky, veggie chips, or cheese crisps to enjoy as a low-carb snack.

Affordable Fats:

Make use of affordable sources of healthful fats, such avocado, butter, and olive oil.

Purchase Meal Preparation Containers:

To portion out meals and cut down on waste, buy reusable meal prep containers.

Examine Cheap Ingredients:

Find affordable Atkins Diet-friendly items including frozen spinach, canned tuna, and cauliflower.

Waste-Free Cooking:

Utilize every portion of your ingredients when cooking to reduce waste. For instance, make homemade broth out of vegetable waste.

Assigning the Task:

If family members or friends are following the Atkins Diet, you might want to pool your resources and buy in bulk to save money.

Accounting Monitoring:

To track how your spending fits with your Atkins Diet journey, keep a budget notebook in which you can record your expenses.

Web-Based Resources:

Discover low-cost Atkins Diet recipes and advice from blogs, forums, and online groups.

Remain Adaptable:

Be flexible and willing to explore new, inexpensive meals and dishes. Accept variety in your diet.

Salute Little Victories:

Whether you're accomplishing your Atkins Diet objectives or staying within your budget, recognize and appreciate your accomplishments.

You may live an affordable Atkins lifestyle and reap the benefits of the diet by following these guidelines and techniques. Remember that you can succeed on the Atkins Diet without going over budget if you have perseverance and creativity.